Ketogenic Diet

Weight Loss Made Easy For Beginners + Quick and Easy at Home Recipes

By Alexander Martin

The trademarks that are used are without any consent, and the publication of the trademark is without permission or backing by the trademark owner. All trademarks and brands within this book are for clarifying purposes only and are owned by the owners themselves, not affiliated with this document.

Table of Contents

Introduction

First off, I want to thank and congratulate you for purchasing the book, *"Ketogenic Diet: Weight Loss Made Easy for Beginners + Quick and Easy at Home Recipes."*

This book contains proven steps and strategies to understand the most important facts about how you can lose weight utilizing and following a ketogenic diet.

Moreover, it explains how a diet that requires the consumption of high fat, moderate protein, and low carbohydrates, can affect not only your weight, but also your overall health. The diet enables the liver to produce ketones that can be utilized by your system instead of glucose in order to give you energy.

This book debunks the common myths regarding the diet. It gives you an idea of what to regularly eat, what you can occasionally indulge in, and what foods you ought to avoid. It also has an entire chapter dedicated to featuring delicious low-carb recipes that are easy to create and modify for you and all your friends.

Thanks again for downloading this book, I hope you enjoy it!

Chapter 1

What is a Ketogenic Diet?

This is the main concept of the ketogenic diet – high fat, moderate protein and low carbohydrate intake. The goal of the diet is to prompt your liver to produce ketones. Through this, your body's metabolisms process will not solely or centrally focus on glucose. Aside from helping you in losing weight, the diet has been proven to be beneficial in many health conditions some of which include: epilepsy, Parkinson's, cancer and Alzheimer's.

When you take in a high dose of carbs, the tendency of your body system is to produce insulin and glucose. Glucose is used by the body as its main source of energy. Insulin is produced in order to regulate the amount of glucose that flows within the bloodstream. Insulin also stores fat in the body. This means that you will gain weight when your body produces too much insulin.

While glucose is known as the primary source of energy that is needed specifically by the brain, it is far from being as efficient as the ketone bodies. Your goal is to introduce your entire system to a dietary shift and in doing so, let it discover how it can manage with having only a little glucose, so that it turns its attention to the ketones for energy.

There are four kinds or varieties of ketogenic diet that you can choose to follow depending on the level of your physical activities and exercise. These are the Standard, Cyclical, Targeted and Restricted. The differences between these four types of the diet depend on the timing of your meals and the daily carb intake. There are numerous studies, which prove that once the body gets keto-adapted, it will run on ketones and automatically stop being dependent on your carb intake before or after exercise.

The focus of the diet is in eating real food. Meaning, you must avoid anything that has additives, artificial sweeteners and preservatives.

How would you know if you are already in the state of ketosis? There are several ways to do this: listen to what your body says, use urine ketone strips, or use a blood ketone meter.

In this kind of diet, it is important that you get your macros or the macronutrient ratio right. Here are the ideal amounts of macros that you should regularly be taking in:

- 65 to 75 percent of calories from fat. This is important so that your body can benefit from the ketone bodies produced by your liver.
- 15 to 30 percent of calories from protein.
- 5 to 10 percent of calories from carbs (net carbs). When you are just starting with the diet, the recommended net carbohydrates that you can intake are from 20 to 30 grams.

It is easier nowadays to track your daily macros. There are various apps that you can download and use for easy reference and macro tracking.

You're now probably asking yourself this question: Is it important to count calories?

If you have been told that you can lose weight even though you do not limit your calorie intake, you have to understand that this is a common misconception. The truth is, it is still possible to gain weight even when you are following a low-carb diet, however the chances are really low.

The ketogenic diet is naturally satisfying. It works by suppressing your appetite, which is the reason why you'll be eating less food. There is no need to count your calorie intake when you are taking in limited food that is able to keep you full.

When should you become alarmed and begin to keep an eye on your calorie intake? Take note of your calorie intake when you have come to a point when or if there are no changes in your weight for more than 3 weeks. This means that you have reached a weight loss plateau.

This plateau can be caused by several factors. It doesn't necessarily mean that you are overeating, but it could actually be because you are not eating enough. As you go about the diet, you will realize that losing weight becomes more difficult when you are already close to your ideal weight.

Is this kind of diet healthy?

Any kind of diet has its pros and cons. You have to listen to your body and observe how it reacts to the dietetic scheme to judge whether or not you should proceed with it. Basically, by being smart with the diet, and by letting your body determine what it needs, you can determine what diet works best for your body.

Many are the health benefits of the diet. We'll explore them in the next chapter.

Chapter 2
Benefits of the Keto Diet

What should you expect when you begin with this kind of a low-carb diet?

Here are some of its health benefits:

Weight Loss – So why does a ketogenic diet lead to successful weight loss? These diets contribute to weight loss for a number of reasons that were previously touched on. However, understanding the details of the weight loss process because of a ketogenic diet is important. First off, the kidneys are able to excrete and filter out excess sodium that is present in the body, which causes weight loss fairly quickly due to the original decrease in insulin levels. Your body will then start burning fat as the main source of energy instead of glucose and as you go into a fasting state, your system will begin to use your fat stores to supply your body with its needed energy.

Emotional Health – Ketone bodies that develop as a result of a ketogenic diet also greatly improve your emotional health and stabilize your mind. This could be because of the production of the inhibitory neurotransmitter, GABA (gamma-amino butyric acid). GABA originates from glutamate, and glutamate itself can become either GABA or aspartate if there is an excess amount of glutamate present in the body. Should there be an excess amount of glutamate in the body, it can cause neurotoxicity within the brain, leading to depression, ALS, migraines, and dementia in some ways, shape, or form. Thankfully, when ketones are metabolized throughout the adoption of the ketogenic diet, they routinely cause glutamate to become GABA instead of aspartate. GABA is a neurotransmitter that is directly involved with the biochemical pathways of divergent mood disorders. For instance, decrease or being deficient in GABA can lead to depression and reduced cognitive function.

Interestingly enough, when studies where done on mitochondria, the organelle of the cell that is in charge of producing the majority of the energy as ATP (adenosine triphosphate), they found that ketone bodies were capable of producing more efficient ATP with fewer waste products. This is extremely important since the brain *craves* clean ATP energy that lacks the presence of free radical waste. By changing the fuel, we are able to alter the levels of GABA and that overall greatly benefits our central nervous system.

Energy – Your body will have a more reliable source of energy. Fats are said to be the most effective molecule to burn for this purpose. You will be pleasantly surprised after you have gotten used to the diet how you are able to remain energetic throughout the day.

Suppresses Hunger – The satisfaction that your body naturally gets from fat leaves you feeling satiated for a longer period of time and prevents feelings of hunger from compromising your weight loss goals.

Helps Fight Cancer Cells – The ketogenic diet could potentially help fight cancer cells in some cases. The theory behind the ability of a low-carbohydrate diet inhibiting the growth and proliferation of cancer cells is quite simple. Since cancer cells require a supply of glucose, than by reducing the amount of glucose present in the body, the cancer cells are unable to receive what they need to survive. It has been discovered that cancer cells function using a different metabolic process in comparison to healthy cells. This means that cancer cells can function well on glucose and fructose and that the primary source of cancer fuel is sugar. That being said, by eating a diet composed mostly of fat you can potentially reduce the growth of cancer cells in the body.

Also, cells comprising cancerous tumors in the body are unable to utilize ketone bodies that are produced following the diet. This is due to the fact that the tumors are unable to respire correctly in the presence of ketone bodies. The importance of this is that you can potentially target the cells of tumors without the excessive use of toxic drugs.

Helps Reduce Seizures – The diet originally gained popularity amongst children and those suffering from epilepsy because it helped diminish seizure frequency. Studies have actually shown that it is able to cause an estimated 50% reduction in the quantity of seizures when children are placed on a strictly followed ketogenic diet. However, when the diet is being followed for the control of seizures, it needs to be carefully monitored and measured by a dietician and medical doctor.

Helps Lower Blood Pressure – Within a matter of days, blood pressure can normalize itself as a result of following the diet. High blood pressure, if not controlled, can lead to the narrowing of blood vessels within the kidneys and the hardening of heart's arteries.

Blood Sugar – As you go along following the diet, you will have less LDL cholesterol, which can effectively get rid of health problems, such as type II diabetes.

Cholesterol – Another benefit of the ketogenic diet is the lowering in cholesterol that takes place. Cholesterol itself is formulated from the excess glucose within the body. In general, cholesterol is a waxy or fatty like substance that is present within the cells that make up the body. The body and all of its cells need cholesterol to function properly; however, if the body has too much cholesterol it can have some serious detrimental side effects. For instance, high cholesterol causes plaque formation and cause arteries to become blocked. Blocked arteries can decrease the amount of blood that is made available to the heart and brain, leading to heart diseases, heart attacks, and strokes to occur. This directly connects to the consumption of less sugar, which occurs naturally when following the diet. Since there is a decrease in the consumption of sugar there is a direct decrease in the amount of damage that occurs within the circulatory system, meaning there is less cholesterol produced.

Prevents Tooth Decay and Gum Disease – Benefits of the ketogenic diet can also be seen in the mouth. Tooth decay and gum disease can be prevented since less sugar is consumed, which creates a change and shift in pH. Because of that, you prevent the formation of periodontitis and stop the gums from pulling away from the teeth and infecting the jawbone.

Healthy Skin – The diet can also help in eliminating acne and overall skin inflammation.

Chapter 3
Identifying Ketosis

Ketosis is a natural metabolic practice by which your body breaks down deposited fat for energy. This may as well result in a dangerous accumulation of ketones in the body known as *ketoacidosis*. Ketosis is regularly the outcome of a low-carbohydrate diet that people make use of in order to lose weight and grow muscle. On the contrary, it can be also be an outcome of malnutrition. Though the enduring risks of ketosis are not clear, there is some indication that it can upsurge your risk of heart disease and developing specific cancers. By identifying the signs of ketosis, you can assist in minimizing your risk for getting ketoacidosis.

Recognizing Signs of Ketosis

1.   **Learn about ketosis.** Doctors understand that ketosis is instigated by an increased level of ketones in the system as a consequence of the body burning fat as fuel. There are specific factors that can place you into a condition of ketosis, which if left abandoned, can grow into the more dangerous condition of ketoacidosis. Ketoacidosis can eventually lead to severe conditions such as brain swelling. Things or risk factors that can put you in a state of ketosis include:

- Being a male
- Consumption of a low carbohydrate diet or in the process of building muscle mass
- Undergoing physical or emotional trauma or stress
- Having diabetes (there is a bigger risk for people

having type I diabetes, but those having type II
diabetes can also experience ketosis)
- Having surgical treatment
- Abusing alcohol and drugs
- Ketoacidosis happens when the levels of ketones
  existing during a ketosis condition rise beyond levels
  that are considered healthy. Ketoacidosis can lead to
  loss of consciousness and even death.

2.   Uncover possible signs of ketosis. There are
some crucial signs connected with ketosis that can assist you
in determining if your body is experiencing this condition.
This can help you in monitoring your level of ketones and
lessen your risk for getting ketoacidosis. The signs of ketosis
consist of:

- Undue or excessive thirst
- Dry mouth, also known as xerostomia
- Reduced appetite
- Strong urine smell do to concentrated waste products
- Feelings of ecstasy or improved energy
- Bad or "fruity"- smelling breath or a metallic taste
  inside your mouth

3.   Note your body functions thoroughly. Because
ketosis can swiftly develop into the dangerous condition of
ketoacidosis, giving close concentration to your body and its
many functions is very vital. This can assist you in getting
timely treatment and can potentially ward off and prevent
bigger problems from occurring.

If you are in ketosis, take note of when the signs begin and
under what situations they stop or cease. Keeping notes may
possibly help you readily detect if you are in ketosis state or
even entering ketoacidosis.

One should keep in mind that the signs of ketosis can differ from one person to another. It can be apparent for some individuals that they are in ketosis state, while on the other hand, other people may not understand what his or her body is experiencing as easily.

4.   Check for ketosis at home. If you presume you are in ketosis state, you can check your belief at home. This can be done by testing urine or measuring blood sugar. Checking these levels substances should be done to ensure that your ketone levels remain healthy.

- You can check ketone levels in your blood using an at-home device. If your blood sugar is above 240mg/dl, you may possibly have too many ketones present within your system.
- You can buy ketone-testing equipment at several pharmacies or medical supply stores. This equipment requires a urine sample, which will change color to indicate or specify the total amount of ketones in your system.
- It's very vital to make use of a dipstick and a clean-catch urine sample to have the most accurate results.

Managing Ketosis

1. **Book an appointment with your doctor.** If you presume your level of ketones are excessively high, book an appointment to discuss your concerns with your doctor. He/she can offer a definitive diagnosis and assist you in formulating an effective plan to continuously monitor your levels of ketones.

- Your doctor may ask for a blood ketone test. This will involve collecting a blood sample from a finger stick or a vein. This may be a more effectual and accurate test than a urinalysis.
- Your doctor may also ask for a urine test to find out the total amount of ketones leaving your system. A downside of this is that it may not be as seamless or precise of a test because it takes time for the ketones to move throughout your entire system.
- Ketoacidosis can eventually bring about problems with your heart, so you may possibly be in need of an electrocardiogram (EKG or ECG) as well.

2. **Manage ketosis.** If your doctor and test results indicate that you are in a ketosis state, he or she may recommend ways to adjust your ketone levels to a healthy and controllable range. This may involve watching and monitoring your diet or undergoing counseling. It is very vital to follow your doctor's recommendations so as to lessen your risk of developing ketoacidosis, which is a very serious condition.

There are quite a few different ways to control the number or quantity of ketones present within your system. These involve: blood sugar monitoring, insulin therapy, and fluid substitution, changing your diet and monitoring hydration.

3.   Desist from workout. If you workout and exercise often, you may want to lessen your energetic activity, if your ketone levels have been found to be above average. Bodybuilding often causes the number of ketones in the body to increase or to experience, "swelling." So that being said, keeping away from bodybuilding type workouts can prevent your ketosis from growing and advancing into ketoacidosis.

If you require some form of activity to assist you in feeling good, think about practicing light activities such as biking or walking, while your ketone levels are above average and on the verge of becoming a healthy level.

4.   Cleanse your system. Staying hydrated is frequently the easiest and most applicable way to keep the level of ketones in your body in check. By drinking plenty of water throughout the day, you may be able to effectively eliminate excessive ketones from your system.

- The majority of people need 9 to 13 cups of water every day, and up to 16 cups if you are living a vigorous lifestyle or are heavy with child.
- Water and other non-caloric drinks are the finest liquids with which to cleanse your system.
- Stay away from drinking too much alcohol or caffeine when your ketones are above average, since these can dehydrate you. As a result of their diuretic properties, they can enhance the amounts of ketones in your system.

5. **Eat a healthy, well-balanced diet.** The majority of people who consume a healthy, well-balanced diet do not encounter enhanced levels of ketones. Eating a low carbohydrate diet in support of a balanced diet can assist you in managing ketone levels and can actually lessen your risk of experiencing or developing ketoacidosis.

- You ought to eat close to 1,800–2,200 calories every day, depending on your individual activity level.
- Acquire calories from a large variety of nutrient-dense whole foods. In your diet involve foods from all of the main food groups: plenty of vegetables and fruits, low-fat dairy, whole grains, and lean proteins. By integrating foods into your diet that you may have normally stayed away from, such as pasta or bread, you may assist yourself in keeping your ketone levels in check.
- Realize that this can potentially cause you gain a little weight, but it's healthier to lessen the risk of ketoacidosis and its associated conditions. It is more important to consume nutritious food than to keep off a couple pounds by staying away from nutrient dense foods.

6. **Control your blood sugar.** If your elevated ketone levels are a result of diabetes or other underlying problems involving your blood sugar, manage it as best as you can by means of both insulin and diet. This may assist you in managing ketone levels and successfully ward off related conditions.

If you are giving yourself insulin injections, your doctor may possibly prescribe a short-term increase in your prescription dosage or the number or quantity of injections you receive on a daily basis.

7.   **Look for counseling.** If you have developed ketosis due to malnutrition or from anorexia nervosa or bulimia, your doctor may possibly refer you to therapy. A therapist can assist you in working through your personal problems with food, which in turn may possibly help in resolving high ketone levels and prevent you from entering ketoacidosis.

If you are lowering carbohydrates to cut weight for any purpose, you may perhaps want to talk it over, with not only your doctor, but also with a therapist. By talking to a therapist you can uncover your motives as to why you may be willing to put your health in danger in exchange for something you personally associate with beauty. Not only that, but therapists can identify and help improve underlying problems with body image.

Ketosis can swiftly become perilous for people suffering from anorexia nervosa or for other people with medical issues. If considering a ketogenic diet plan, talk to your doctor and acquire an approved medical diet plan before starting your new diet. Be sure to follow health and diet rules to care for your well-being and to help keep your ketone levels within a healthy range.

Chapter 4
Debunking the Myths about the Ketogenic Diet

Is a ketogenic diet effective in helping you lose weight or is it just another fad diet that will lose popularity in a short span of time? It is both an effective and healthy diet. It offers many benefits aside from just weight loss, and all of this diets many claims are backed up with scientific studies and research.

Just like any diet, it does not work in the same mechanism for everybody, but it does not necessarily mean that it will harm you. The following are the most common myths about this low-carbohydrate diet that you must not fall for:

1. It is restrictive and hard to sustain.

Come to think of it, all diets restrict something. The good thing about carbohydrate restriction is that it suppresses your appetite. You will eat until you are full, so you will not feel like you are being deprived of food or energy. This is far from a low-calorie diet wherein food is limited and you end up feeling hungry and lacking energy most of the time.

2. It does more harm than good for your heart.

Many people fear the inclusion of too much fat in the diet and automatically associate this with the increased risk of heart disease. This low-carb diet prompts you to eat saturated fat and dietary cholesterol that do not have any significant effect on your risk of heart problems. It actually works the other way around because it reduces your chances of developing heart ailments due to the following:

- It boosts the level of your good cholesterol, known as HDL.
- It reduces your blood triglycerides.
- It decreases resistance to insulin, which in effect will lower your insulin and blood sugar levels.
- It lowers your risk for inflammation throughout your system.

3. Ketosis is not healthy and is bad for your health.

Many people incorrectly think ketosis and ketoacidosis are interchangeable. These two are not the same. Ketosis is a healthy metabolic state, while ketoacidosis is dangerous and is often experienced by those who have uncontrolled type I diabetes. What makes ketoacidosis harmful? Ketoacidosis floods your bloodstream with too many ketones, which make the pH of the blood drop and become acidic. It can be fatal if not controlled.

Ketosis has nothing to do with ketoacidosis. Ketosis can even help in treating epilepsy and is now being studied for its positive effects in treating brain diseases and cancer.

When you take in less than 50 grams of carbs each day, the tendency is for your insulin levels to decrease and for high amounts of fat to get released from the fat cells. The fatty acids travel to the liver and get turned into ketones or ketone bodies. Ketones are molecules that can pass through the blood brain barrier and enter the brain as to supply it energy at times when you eat low amounts of carbs.

4. This kind of diet only reduces your water weight.

When you consume too many carbohydrates, most of them are stored in the liver and muscles. Glucose or glycogen (the storage form of glucose) is formed from this storage. The stored glycogen in your muscles and liver binds a certain amount of water. When you take in fewer carbohydrates, the tendency is for the stored glycogen to decrease, which leads to the loss of significant amounts of water weight.

Low-carb diets lead to a drastic decrease in the levels of your insulin. As a result, your kidneys will eliminate excess water and sodium from your body. These diets cause a decrease in water weight, but most of the weight loss comes from the reduction in body fat, especially in the abdominal area and liver. Losing water weight is not a bad thing because it is only representative of the excess weight that you are carrying.

5. The brain cannot function without glucose that is obtained from carbs.

There are some cells in the brain that can only function using glucose as fuel. Most parts of the brain are capable of running using ketones as fuel. When you consume fewer carbohydrates to prompt ketosis, the majority of the brain stops being solely dependent on glucose and instead turns to ketones for fuel.

Where will the body get the glucose that is needed by some parts of the brain? It is not necessary to consume carbohydrates for the mere purpose of fueling the brain. Glucose can be produced through the metabolic pathway that is known as gluconeogenesis, the new formation of glucose.

When your body does not receive enough carbs from the diet, the liver and the rest of the system take charge in producing glucose from the protein and the by-products of the metabolism of fat. Your body will take time to adjust to the changes occurring and after the initial adaptation phase, the brain will be able to function better.

6. Low-carb diet makes you weak and will affect your physical performance.

Many people who are into heavy physical activities eat high amounts of carbohydrates. Part of the initial setback of a low-carb diet is the reduced performance some people may experience, but this is only temporary. If you give your body enough time to adjust to burning fat instead of carbs and you will go back to your usual routine in a short amount of time.

Chapter 5
Learning Which Foods to Eat and Which to Avoid

The most important thing that you need to remember when following the ketogenic diet is that you must eat real food. Avoid processed foods and anything that has added color, dyes, and preservatives. More importantly, besides losing weight, the keto diet helps you in developing a healthy routine. It is not only a diet, but also rather more like a healthy lifestyle.

Foods to Eat

1. Healthy fats

- Saturated – butter, ghee, coconut oil, chicken fat, clarified butter, lard, tallow, goose fat and duck fat
- Monounsaturated – olive oil, avocado oil and macadamia oil
- Polyunsaturated omega-3 fatty acids – seafood and fatty fish

2. Wild and grass-fed animal sources

- Wild-caught fish and seafood
- Grass-fed meat – lamb, venison, goat and beef
- Pastured eggs
- Pastured pork and poultry
- Offal from grass-fed animals – organ meats that include kidneys, liver and heart

3. Nuts, seeds and fruits

- Macadamia nuts
- Coconut
- Avocado

4. Non-starchy vegetables

- Cruciferous vegetables – radishes, dark leaf kale, kohlrabi
- Asparagus, summer squash (spaghetti squash, zucchini), cucumber, celery stalk and bamboo shoots
- Leafy greens – bok choy, Swiss chard, chard, spinach, radicchio, lettuce, endive, chives, etc.

5. Beverages and Condiments

- Water, black tea, herbal tea, black coffee, coffee with cream or coconut milk
- Herbs and spices, lime or lemon juice and zest
- Utilization of pork rinds for breading
- Bone broth, mustard, mayonnaise, pickles, pesto, fermented foods like sauerkraut, kimchi and kombucha
- Gelatin, whey protein and egg white (albumen) protein

Foods that You Can Eat Occasionally

1. Dairy and animal sources that are grain-fed

- Eggs, poultry, ghee and beef
- Bacon (Be sure not buy anything with added starches and preservatives.)
- Dairy products (Avoid buying products that are labeled as "low-fat." Most of them contain excess

starch and sugar.) – plain full-fat yogurt, cheese, cream, sour cream and cottage cheese

2. Mushrooms, vegetables and fruits

- Spring onion, mushrooms, onion, garlic, winter squash (pumpkin) and leek
- Some cruciferous vegetables – red cabbage, white and green cabbage, fennel, cauliflower, turnips, Brussels sprouts, rutabaga and broccoli
- Bean, okra and sea vegetables, such as kombu and nori
- Nightshades, such as tomatoes, eggplant and peppers
- Sugar snap peas, sprouts, water chestnuts and wax beans
- Olives, rhubarb and berries, such as blueberries, raspberries, blackberries, mulberries, cranberries, strawberries, etc.

3. Fermented soy products

- Unprocessed black soybeans and edamame or green soy beans
- Soy sauce, Tempeh, Natto, Paleo-friendly coconut aminos

4. Seeds and nuts

- Brazil nuts (Be sure to eat these in moderation because they contain high amounts of selenium)

- Almonds, pumpkin seeds, pecans, sunflower seeds, walnuts, hemp seeds, pine nuts, sesame seeds, hazelnuts and flaxseed

5. Condiments

- Sugar-free tomato products – Ketchup, puree, passata
- Thickeners – xanthan gum, arrowroot powder
- Zero-carb sweeteners that are healthy – Stevia, Erythritol, Swerve
- Extra dark chocolate (more than 70 percent cacao), carob powder and cocoa

6. Certain nuts, fruits, seeds, and vegetables containing average carbs

- Chestnuts, pistachios, and cashew nuts
- Peach, apricot, dragon fruit, watermelon, orange, fresh figs, kiwi berries, kiwifruit, plums, apple, nectarine, grapefruit
- Dried fruits, such as raisins, berries, figs and dates
- Root vegetables, such as carrots, sweet potato, celery root, parsnip and beetroot

7. Alcohol

- Dry white wine
- Unsweetened spirits
- Dry red wine

Foods that You Must Completely Avoid

1. Processed foods, especially the types that contain the following:

- MSG
- BPAs
- Carrageenan
- Wheat gluten
- Sulphites

2. Factory-farmed fish and pork

3. Artificial sweeteners

- Sweeteners that contain Aspartame, Sucralose, Saccharin and Acesulfame
- Equal, Splenda

4. Grains

- Whole meal – oats, wheat, rice, sorghum, barley, corn, rye, sprouted grains, bulgur, millet, buckwheat, amaranth
- White potatoes and quinoa
- Products that are made from grains – bread, cookies, pasta, crackers and pizza

5. Sugar and sweets

- Ice cream
- Table sugar
- Agave syrup
- Soft drinks

- Cakes

6. Tropical fruits

- Mango
- Papaya
- Pineapple
- Banana

7. High-carb fruits

- Grapes
- Tangerine

8. Refined oils and fats

- Canola
- Corn oil
- Sunflower
- Cottonseed
- Safflower
- Soybean
- Trans fats (margarine)

9. Milk –Try and only allow yourself to take small amounts of full-fat and raw milk.

10. Sweet alcoholic drinks

- Cocktails
- Beer

- Sweet wine

Chapter 6
Easy-to-Do Ketogenic Recipes

Sample Breakfast Recipes

Keto-Friendly Blueberry Ricotta Pancakes

Yield: 5 servings

Nutritional info per serving: 13.4 grams of protein, 22.6 grams of fats, 296.6 calories, and 5.9 grams net carbs

Ingredients:

- 1 cup of almond flour
- 3 eggs
- 1/2 cup of golden flaxseed meal
- 1 teaspoon of baking powder
- 3/4 cup of ricotta
- 1/4 teaspoon of salt
- 1/2 teaspoon vanilla extract
- 1/4 cup of blueberries
- 1/4 cup of unsweetened vanilla almond milk
- 1/2 teaspoon of stevia powder

Directions:

1. Put the eggs, almond milk, ricotta and vanilla extract in a blender. Process until well-combined.

2. In a bowl, put the almond flour, baking powder, salt, stevia and golden flaxseed meal, and mix. Transfer this to the blender that contains the previously made egg mixture. Process until the consistency is that of a smooth batter.

3. Melt butter in a skillet over medium heat. Pour 2 tablespoons of the batter for each serving and add 2 to 3 blueberries. Cook both sides.

4. Serve the pancakes with sugar-free syrup and add some berries on top.

Keto White Pizza Frittata

Yield: 8 servings

Nutritional info per serving: 19.4 grams of protein, 23.8 grams of fats, 298 calories, and 2.1 grams net carbs

Ingredients:

- 4 tablespoons of olive oil
- 12 eggs
- 1 ounce of pepperoni
- 1 teaspoon of minced garlic
- 1/2 cup of Parmesan cheese
- 1/2 cup of fresh ricotta cheese
- 5 ounces of mozzarella cheese
- 9-ounce bag of frozen spinach (thawed and drained)
- 1/4 teaspoon of nutmeg
- Salt and pepper

Directions:

1. Mix the eggs, spices, and olive oil in a bowl. Add the spinach (broken into small pieces), ricotta, and Parmesan. Transfer this into a cast iron skillet. Sprinkle the mozzarella cheese and arrange the pepperoni on top.

2. Bake in a preheated oven at 375 degrees for 30 minutes. Slice and serve.

Healthy Breakfast Burger

Yield: 2 servings

Nutritional info per serving: 30.5 grams of protein, 56 grams of fats, 655 calories, and 3 grams net carbs

Ingredients:

- 4 slices of bacon
- 4 ounces of sausage
- 2 eggs
- 2 ounces of Pepperjack cheese
- 1 tablespoon of PB Fit Powder
- 1 tablespoon of butter
- Salt and pepper

Directions:

1. Cook the bacon in an oven at 400 degrees for 25 minutes.

2. In a small bowl, combine the PB Fit powder and butter. Set aside.

3. Form and cook 2 sausage patties until well-done. Put cheese on top of each patty, cover the pan, and remove from heat.

4. Cook the eggs.

5. Assemble your burger and serve immediately.

Pumpkin Pie Spice Latte

Yield: 3 servings

Nutritional info per serving: 0.4 gram of protein, 13 grams of fats, 132 calories, and 2.1 grams net carbs

Ingredients:

- 2 cups of strong, freshly brewed coffee
- 2 tablespoons of heavy whipping cream
- 1 cup of coconut milk
- 2 tablespoons of butter
- 1/4 cup of pumpkin puree
- 15 drops of liquid stevia
- 2 teaspoons of pumpkin pie spice blend
- 1/2 teaspoon of cinnamon
- 1 teaspoon of vanilla extract

Directions:

1. In a saucepan over medium heat, mix the butter, milk, pumpkin, and spices. Once the mixture starts bubbling, add the brewed coffee and mix well. Remove from the stove.

2. Put the stevia and cream into the mixture. Use an immersion blender to combine all ingredients.

3. Serve with whipped cream on top.

Sample Recipes for Lunch

Sausage and Kale Soup

Yield: 6 servings

Nutritional info per serving: 16 grams of protein, 24 grams of fats, 298 calories, and 6 grams net carbs

Ingredients:

- 1 pound of ground sweet Italian sausage
- 1 carrot (peeled and diced)
- 1 yellow onion (chopped)
- 1 tablespoon of butter
- 2 tablespoons of red wine vinegar
- 2 cloves of garlic (crushed)
- 1 cup of heavy cream
- 4 cups of low-sodium chicken broth
- 3 cups of kale (chopped)
- 1/2 teaspoon of crushed red pepper flakes
- Sea salt and freshly ground black pepper to taste
- 1/2 of cauliflower (cut into small florets)
- 1 teaspoon of each of the following: dried rubbed sage, dried oregano, and dried basil

Directions:

1. Cook the sausage in a saucepan over medium-high heat. Stir occasionally, break up the meat, and continue cooking until the meat browns. Transfer the cooked sausage on a

plate lined with paper towels. Discard the drippings from the pan.

2. Adjust the heat of the stove to medium. Put butter in the pan. Once the butter melts, cook the carrots and onions for 3 minutes. Add the garlic while stirring and continue to cook for 1 minute. Add the red wine vinegar and cook for 1 more minute. Next, add the red pepper flakes, herbs, heavy cream, and chicken broth. Turn the heat to medium-high. Wait for the soup to simmer.

3. Turn the heat to medium-low and add the cauliflower florets. Simmer for an additional 10 minutes. Finally, add the cooked sausage and kale, and cook for a couple of minutes. Season with salt and pepper as needed.

Broccoli Chicken Zucchini Boats

Yield: 2 servings

Nutritional info per serving: 30 grams of protein, 34 grams of fats, and 5 grams net carbs

Ingredients:

- 1 cup of broccoli florets (cut into small pieces)
- 2 large zucchinis
- 6 ounces of rotisserie chicken (shredded)
- 2 tablespoons of butter
- 1 stalk of green onion
- 3 ounces of cheddar cheese (shredded)
- 2 tablespoons of sour cream
- Salt and pepper to taste

Directions:

1. Cut the zucchini in half lengthwise. Scoop out the pulp until there is about a 1 cm thickness left for the shell. Put a tablespoon of melted butter into each shell. Season with salt and pepper. Bake in an oven preheated at 400 degrees for 20 minutes.

2. In a bowl, mix the broccoli, shredded chicken, and sour cream. Season with salt and pepper accordingly. Put the filling in each baked zucchini. Sprinkle with cheddar cheese. Bake for 15 more minutes.

3. Serve with a dollop of sour cream and garnish with chopped green onion.

Keto Mixed Green Spring Salad

Yield: 1 serving

Nutritional info per serving: 17.1 grams of protein, 37.3 grams of fats, 478 calories, and 4.3 grams net carbs

Ingredients:

- 2 slices of bacon
- 2 ounces of mixed greens
- 2 tablespoons of shredded Parmesan cheese
- 2 tablespoons of low-carb raspberry vinaigrette
- 3 tablespoons of pine nuts (roasted)
- Salt and pepper to taste

Directions:

1. Cook the bacon in a pan until crisp. Allow cooling before crumbling the cooked bacon slices.

2. Put the crumbled bacon in a bowl along with the rest of the ingredients. Mix well and serve.

Keto Grilled Cheese Sandwich

Yield: 1 serving

Nutritional info per serving: 29 grams of protein, 70 grams of fats, 793 calories, and 4.7 grams net carbs

Ingredients:

For the bun:

- 2 tablespoons of almond flour
- 2 eggs
- 2 tablespoons of butter (room temperature)
- 1 1/2 tablespoons of psyllium husk powder
- 1/2 teaspoon of baking powder

For the filling and extras:

- 2 ounces of cheddar cheese
- 1 tablespoon of butter (for frying)

Directions:

1. Put all of the ingredients for the bun in a single bowl. Mix well until thick. Transfer the mixture into a square container. Microwave for 90 seconds. Add more time, if needed, until the mixture is cooked. Remove from the container and slice in half.

2. Arrange the sandwich by placing cheese in the middle of the bun that was just made. Put butter in a heated pan. Fry the sandwich until browned.

Sample Recipes for Dinner

Skillet Browned Chicken with Creamy Greens

Yield: 4 servings

Nutritional info per serving: 18.42 grams of protein, 38.19 grams of fats, 446 calories, and 2.61 grams net carbs

Ingredients:

- 1 cup of chicken stock
- 1 cup of cream
- 1 pound of chicken thighs (boneless)
- 2 cups of dark leafy greens
- 2 tablespoons of coconut flour
- 2 tablespoons of coconut oil
- 2 tablespoons of melted butter
- 1 teaspoon of Italian herbs
- Salt and pepper to taste

Directions:

1. Put coconut oil in a pan on medium-high heat.

2. Rub the chicken thighs with salt and pepper. Put it in the pan and cook both sides until crispy.

3. Work on the sauce while the chicken is cooking. Put 2 tablespoons of butter in a small saucepan and cook over low heat. Once the butter melts, add 2 tablespoons of coconut flour and whisk. Add a cup of cream, stir, and bring to a boil. Once the mixture becomes thick, add the herbs and stir.

4. Transfer the cooked chicken to a plate. Place the chicken stock into the pan to deglaze it. Transfer the cream sauce to the same pan. Add the greens and stir until they are coated with the sauce. Place the chicken directly on top of the sauce mixture. Remove from the stove.

5. Serve and enjoy.

Creamy Crab Zucchini Casserole

Yield: 9 servings

Nutritional info per serving: 7.2 grams of protein, 11.9 grams of fats, 162.6 calories, and 2.8 grams net carbs

Ingredients:

- 3 zucchini squash (spiralized using the wide ribbon setting)
- Butter (for greasing)
- 1 tablespoon of butter
- 4 ounces of cream cheese (chunked)
- 1/2 cup of heavy cream
- 1 tablespoon of red wine vinegar
- 2 teaspoons of "Old Bay" seasoning
- 1 clove of garlic (crushed)
- 1 onion (halved and sliced)
- 8 ounces of crab meat
- 1/2 cup of Mexican blend cheese (finely grated)
- 3 green onions (thinly sliced)
- Salt and pepper to taste

Directions:

1. Season the spiralized zucchini with salt before steaming for 7 minutes or until zucchini is tender.

2. Melt the butter in a skillet over medium heat. Add the onions and cook until tender. Next, add the garlic and cook for 1 minute. Proceed to add the vinegar. Stir until most of the vinegar has evaporated. Put the cream cheese and cream

into the skillet. Continue cooking while frequently stirring until the cheese has melted. Put the green onion, crab meat and "Old Bay" seasoning into the skillet with the previously added ingredients. Season with salt and pepper. Add the zucchini and mix well.

3. Transfer the dish to a 9x9 baking dish that has been greased with butter. Sprinkle grated cheese on top. Bake in a preheated oven at 375 degrees for 25 minutes

4. Serve and enjoy.

Keto-Friendly Sushi

Yield: 3 servings

Nutritional info per serving (1 1/2 rolls): 18.3 grams of protein, 25.7 grams of fats, 353 calories, and 5.7 grams net carbs

Ingredients:

- 5 sheets of nori
- Half of a medium avocado
- A single 6-inch cucumber
- 5 ounces of smoked salmon
- 16 ounces of cauliflower
- 6 ounces of cream cheese (softened)
- 1 tablespoon of soy sauce
- 2 tablespoons of rice vinegar (unseasoned)

Directions:

1. Put the cauliflower in a food processor. Pulse until the consistency is similar to rice.

2. Slice each end of the cucumber. Place it upright and slice off each side. Discard the middle seeded portion. Continue to slice the 2 side parts into thin strips. Place in the fridge.

3. Cook the cauliflower rice in a pan over medium-high heat. Add about a tablespoon of soy sauce. Remove from the stove.

4. Put the cauliflower "rice" in a bowl and mix with rice vinegar and cream cheese. Mix well and refrigerate.

5. Scoop out the avocado from the shell and cut into small strips.

6. Lay a nori sheet on a bamboo roller that is lined with saran wrap. Spread an even layer of the cauliflower rice. Put the other fillings on top of the cauliflower rice, and roll in a tight manner. Slice and serve.

Low-Carb Pumpkin Carbonara

Yield: 3 servings

Nutritional info per serving: 14 grams of protein, 34.7 grams of fats, 384 calories, and 2 grams net carbs

Ingredients:

- 5 ounces of pancetta (chopped)
- 2 egg yolks
- 1 package of shirataki noodles
- 2 tablespoons of butter
- 1/4 cup of heavy cream
- 1/2 teaspoon of dried sage
- 1/3 cup of Parmesan cheese
- 3 tablespoons of pumpkin puree
- Salt and pepper to taste

Directions:

1. Immerse the noodles in hot water for 3 minutes. Drain and allow them to dry completely. Set aside.

2. Put the pancetta in a pan over medium-high heat. Cook until crisp. Transfer to a plate and be sure to save the fat.

3. Put butter in a small pan over medium heat and allow to brown. Put the pumpkin puree and sage into the small pan. Mix well. Add the pancetta fat and heavy cream. Stir until well-combined. Add the Parmesan cheese. Turn the heat to low. Mix until the sauce becomes thick.

4. Put the shirataki noodles in the pan where you cooked the pancetta. Dry fry for 5 minutes.

5. Put the pancetta and noodles into the sauce. Mix and toss. Add the egg yolks and continue mixing.

Recipe Ideas for Dessert

No Bake Coconut Cashew Bars

Yield: 8 servings

Nutritional info per serving: 4 grams of protein, 17.6 grams of fats, 189 calories, and 4 grams net carbs

Ingredients:

- 1 cup of almond flour
- 1/4 cup of maple syrup (sugar-free)
- 1/4 cup of melted butter
- 1/2 cup of cashews (chopped)
- 1/4 cup of shredded coconut
- 1 teaspoon of cinnamon
- A pinch of salt

Directions:

1. In a bowl, place the almond flour and melted butter. Mix until well-combined. Add the shredded coconut, salt, cinnamon, cashews and maple syrup. Mix well.

2. Spread the dough in a baking dish that is lined with parchment paper. Chill in the refrigerator for a few hours. Slice into bars and serve.

Pumpkin Pecan Pie Ice Cream

Yield: 4 servings

Nutritional info per serving (1 cup): 6.5 grams of protein, 22.3 grams of fats, 248 calories, and 4.3 grams net carbs

Ingredients:

- 1/2 cup of pumpkin puree
- 1 teaspoon of pumpkin spice
- 2 cups of coconut milk
- 1/2 cup of cottage cheese
- 20 drops of liquid stevia
- 3 egg yolks
- 1/3 cup of Erythritol
- 1/2 teaspoon of Xanthan gum
- 2 tablespoons of salted butter
- 1/2 cup of toasted pecans (chopped)
- 1 teaspoon of maple extract

Directions:

1. Melt butter in a pan, add the toasted pecans and stir.

2. Put the remaining ingredients into a blender and process until a smooth constancy is reached. Transfer the mixture into an ice cream machine. Add the pecans with the butter from step 1. Allow the machine to churn according to instructions.

Recipe Ideas for Snacks

Pesto Keto Crackers

Yield: 6 servings

Nutritional info per serving: 5 grams of protein, 20 grams of fats, 210 calories, and 3 grams net carbs

Ingredients:

- 1 1/4 cups of almond flour
- 1/2 teaspoon of baking powder
- 1 clove of garlic (pressed)
- 1/2 teaspoon of salt
- 1/4 teaspoon of ground black pepper
- 2 tablespoons of basil pesto
- 1/4 teaspoon of dried basil
- 3 tablespoons of butter
- A pinch of cayenne pepper

Directions:

1. In a bowl, put the flour, baking powder, salt, and pepper. Whisk in order to combine ingredients until smooth. Put the pressed garlic, basil, and cayenne into the bowl. Mix well. Add the pesto. Continue whisking until the dough appears to look like coarse crumbs. Add the butter and cut it into the mixture using a fork. Form the dough into a ball.

2. Spread the dough thinly on a cookie sheet lined with parchment paper. Bake in a preheated oven at 325 degrees for 17 minutes or until golden brown.

3. Remove from the oven and cut the crackers into your preferred sizes.

Raspberry Lemon Popsicles

Yield: 6 servings

Nutritional info per serving: 0.5 gram of protein, 16 grams of fats, 151 calories, and 2 grams net carbs

Ingredients:

- 100 grams of raspberries
- 1 cup of coconut milk
- Juice from 1/2 lemon
- 1/4 cup of sour cream
- 1/4 cup of coconut oil
- 1/2 teaspoon of guar gum
- 1/4 cup of heavy cream
- 20 drops of liquid stevia

Directions:

1. Put all of the ingredients into a bowl. Blend using an immersion blender. Strain to discard any of the raspberry seeds.

2. Pour the popsicle mixture into molds. Chill for a couple of hours in the freezer.

3. Remove the popsicles from the molds. Serve and enjoy.

No-Bake Peanut Butter Chocolate Fat Bombs

Yield: 8 servings

Nutritional info per serving: 4.4 grams of protein, 20 grams of fats, 208 calories, and 0.8 gram net carbs

Ingredients:

- 2 tablespoons of heavy cream
- 1/4 cup of cocoa powder
- 6 tablespoons of shelled hemp seeds
- 28 drops of liquid stevia
- 4 tablespoons of PB Fit powder
- 1/2 cup of coconut oil
- 1/4 cup of unsweetened shredded coconut
- 1 teaspoon of vanilla extract

Directions:

1. Mix all of the dry ingredients in a bowl. Add the coconut oil. Mix well until it turns into a paste. Add the liquid stevia, heavy cream, and vanilla. Mix thoroughly until slightly creamy.

2. Spread out the unsweetened shredded coconut on a plate.

3. Form the dough into small balls. Roll each ball on the plate with the shredded coconut so that the ball becomes covered in coconut. Arrange the finished pieces on a tray that is lined with parchment paper. Chill for 20 minutes before serving.

Conclusion

Thank you again for reading this book!

I hope this book was able to help you understand what the ketogenic diet is all about and how it can help you in losing weight and living a healthy lifestyle.

The next step to following this diet is to stock up on all of the right ingredients so you can plan your meals, and begin with the diet as soon as you can.

Finally, if you enjoyed this book or found it helpful, I would ask that you would be kind enough to **leave a review** for this book on Amazon. It would be greatly appreciated!

Thank you and good luck in becoming the healthiest and best-looking version of yourself! ☺

Check Out My Other Book

Below you'll find a link to my other popular book on Amazon and Kindle.

<u>Intermittent Fasting: Burn Fat, Lose Weight & Be The Best Version of Yourself</u>

Check Out Our Blog

<u>http://www.physicalpower.fit</u>

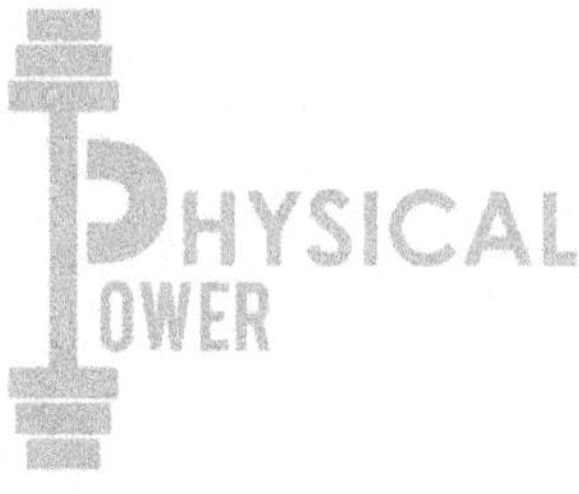